# Also by Dr. Stenbeck

## Available from the usual on-line source

### Books

Healing Yourself -- The Holistic Approach
[An introduction to Holistic Self-healing.]

Heal Yourself Right Now!
[The Seven Priority Organ Levels for
effective Nutritional/Holistic Treatment of
all organs.]

**The 22 Unique Body Types**
(for Health and Weight Loss)

Q & A to Identify Your Body Type (Booklet)
[Individual Type booklets are also available

### Booklets
(Step-by-step instructions on healing yourself)

#1 Start Healing with Positive Thinking
#2 Mastering Positive Feelings for Health!
#3 Spiritual Balance and Your Healing

# The Atrophic Body Type

*Representing one of the 22 Body Types first described by Victor Rocine around 1900*

---

## The Woody Allen, Calista Flockheart Celebrity Body Type

*For Kaye,*
*there at the beginning with Doc Severn,*
*and for Liberty,*
*continuing the holistic healing journey…*

# Disclaimer

The information in this book is for educational purposes only and is not a substitute for medication, diets, or other medical care. The diets do not treat diseases or medical conditions, and are an adjunct to your orthodox health care.

The author and publisher accept no responsibility for any misuse of the information within. If you have any physical problem, food allergy, emotional disorder, or disease, common sense dictates that you consult with a physician before changing your diet, taking nutritional supplements, or following the advice given here.

———

# About the Author

Educated in New Zealand and in the U.S.A., Dr. Stenbeck attained B.Sc. (NZ), M.S., and D.C. degrees. His holistic healing methods have been profiled in magazines (Esquire, McLean's, Playgirl, the Atlanta Constitution), and on TV in the USA and in Canada. He was the main contributor to the Warner Book by Jessica Maxwell, _The Eye/Body Connection,_ that focused on the holistic healing relationships between the iris structure and organ genetics.

In the 1970-80's he was elected Fellow, Royal Society of Health, London; Fellow, American Association of Chemists; Member, American Association of Clinical Chemists; and Affiliate, Royal Society of Medicine, London. He studied naturopathy and Body Types with Dr. Bernard Jensen and Dr. Clifford Severn, and has practiced in medical partnerships where patients received the joint benefits of medical and holistic healing.

He is a member of Self-Realization Fellowship. To receive advice on any health issue from a holistic viewpoint, or to receive help with your body type, see his web site: *DrStenbeck.net*

———

# Contents

\* \* \*

The 22 Body Types with Celebrity Examples    x
A Succinct Quote from Victor Rocine    xiii
Prologue    xiv

## The Atrophic Body Type and Food Guide    1

## Appendix

A. Types /Minerals    48
B. Researchers    52
C. Genetics, Types, and Diet    54
D. Help identifying your body type with
    Dr. Stenbeck    57
E. On-line health consultation with
    Dr. Stenbeck    60
F. Notes    61

# The 22 Body Types:
## Celebrity Examples

---

*This Booklet contains the **Atrophic** type. See The 22 Unique Body Types for all type descriptions.]*

---

## Thin Types

| | |
|---|---|
| **Atrophic** | *Woody Allen / Audrey Hepburn*<br>*Stan Laurel / Calista Flockheart* |
| *Exesthesic* | *Cher / Sarah Jessica Parker*<br>*(Female type only)* |
| *Marasmic* | *President Obama / Princess Diana*<br>*James Stewart / Kate Blanchard* |
| *Neurogenic* | *J.K. Simmons / Joan Rivers*<br>*Jon Cryer / Marin Hinle* |
| *Pathoferic* | *(No celebrity males)*<br>*Blythe Danner / Gwyneth Paltrow* |
| *Sillevitic* | *David Bowie / Shirley MacLaine*<br>*Rod Stewart / Carol Channing* |

---

## Muscle Types

Calciferic     Michael Jordan / Angelica Huston
               Abraham Lincoln / Grace Jones

Carbogenic     George Clooney / Lady Gaga
               Pres. G. Bush, Jr. / Meg Ryan

Desmogenic     Marlon Brando / Loni Anderson
               Daniel Craig / Tina Turner

Eldic          Ross Perot / Hillary Clinton
               Peter Falk / Sigourney Weaver

Myogenic       Pres. Bill Clinton / Sharon Stone
               Pres. John Kennedy / Julia Roberts

Nervimotive    Frank Sinatra / Elizabeth Taylor
               Mark Wahlberg / Natalie Wood

Nitropheric    Ben Affleck / Ava Gardner
               Kirk Douglas / Kate Winslet

Pallinomic     Pres. Donald Trump /
               Attorney General Janet Reno
               Bill O'Reilly (Fox) / Jane Russell

---

## *Fat Types*

*Barotic*          *Robin Williams / 'Mrs.Doubtfire'*
                      *Elton John / William Conrad*

*Carboferic*      *Bill Murray / Roseanne*
                      *Billy Gardell / Melissa McCarthy*

*Hydripheric*    *John Goodman / Shelly Winters*
                      *Wayne Knight / Jennifer Holliday*

*Isogenic*         *Einstein / Oprah Winfrey*
                      *Phillip S .Hoffman / Queen Victoria*

*Lipopheric*      *Rush Limbaugh / Rosie O'Donnell*
                      *Chris Christie / Camryn Manheim*

*Oxypheric*      *Winston Churchill / Orsen Welles*
                      *Ella Fitzgerald / Gerry Spence*

*Pargenic*        *Burt Reynolds / Katey Segal*
                      *Ron Perlman / Kirstey Alley*

---

## *Succinct Quote on Human Types*

*From Victor Rocine, who first described discrete body types around 1900.*

"A type is an order of people that differentiates and distinguishes itself by a general and similar form, brain-formation, chemistry, structure, build, immunity, tendencies, predisposition, resemblance, skin-pigment, and type characteristics based on observation and analogy.

"Or, in other words, people of a given type are similar physically and like-minded as if they were brothers and sisters—that is what type means.

"Everything in nature is made according to plan. Man only discovers that plan and gives it a name. The zoologist has not made the animals—he has only described the plan adopted by the wonderful Creator, and named the classes, sub-classes, etc.

"How important type research will be to humanity, time alone will make known."

———

# *Prologue*

The esteemed scientist J. J. Berzelius, discoverer of several chemical elements, inspired Victor Rocine to research body types and to investigate the correlation between types and their diseases. Around 1890-1910, Rocine privately published his original findings on the mineral basis of different body types, and this present book exists because of his brilliant insights.

For many years, I studied with Dr. Clifford Severn who had been a personal student of Victor Rocine on body types, naturopathy, herbology, iris analysis, diet, and nutritional healing methods. He had a successful career as a lecturer and healer, and was one of those rare athletes with complete muscle control over his body. I saw him under a spotlight at 85 years of age, contracting and rippling every individual muscle in his perfectly developed body. Field-Marshal Jan Smuts, the WWII South African Prime Minister, devoted a full chapter of his autobiography to how Severn's healing methods had saved his life. In the 1950's, *Life* magazine did a four-page spread on Severn and his family. Fame he had.

Another Rocine student I studied with, Dr. Bernard Jensen wrote of Rocine's body type research and nutritional methods in his privately published book *The Chemistry of Man*.

This book is deeply rooted in Rocine's original work, and with that of Herbert Shelton, M.D., Ph.D. (at Harvard University in the 1930's). I integrated their research with newer dietary and nervous system data along with celebrity examples of each type, hopefully, making this material easier to digest and more entertaining for the reader.

Gayelord Hauser, another Rocine student I knew, was a celebrated health book author. He wrote a popular book on Rocine's types in the 1940's, *Types and Temperaments;* reputedly, he also introduced yogurt to the western world.

This book exists because of Rocine's creative brilliance and original discoveries in natural healing.

▶ *Rocine: "The soul creates the body type."*

Rocine taught that the soul chooses a body type and brain to live in, thus presenting different experiences and life lessons to master. Why were *you* born the way you are?

That is something to think about, especially if it is true! What would your soul purpose be to live in a particular body type. I provide some thoughts on this issue in each type description and try to assess from my experience with your type the particular lessons of life presented therein.

Rocine was as brilliant in his way as an Abraham Lincoln, Michael Jordan, Michael Phelps, Tony Robbins, or a Daniel Day Lewis—all *calciferic* types—rare, leaders, innovative, brilliant, and highly intelligent in their different fields of endeavor.

Celebrity examples exist for most types, not a duplicate of you, but someone who has your essence in their body-mind individuality. Knowing your type allows you to become a better you!

The celebrity examples provide further help in identifying your body type.

▶ *Rocine's classic findings are the backbone of this book. Integrated with Sheldon's research and with other dietary and food issues including mental, emotional, and spiritual attributes,*

Many people take nutritional supplements and try different diets without a doctor's advice. If this is your choice, use common sense, listen to body responses, and discontinue any allergic reactions to foods or nutritional substances.

———

# The Atrophic Body Type

*** 

*"You may also have a physical or psychological feature not representative of your type such as height, weight, appearance, talent, weakness, strength, etc., due to biochemical errors, environmental influences, racial or cultural differences, and congenital or genetic issues. Nevertheless, the type identification of the average person is usually clear."*

— *Victor Rocine*

# *The Atrophic Type Celebrity Examples*

*If you think this is your type, be sure to look at* **on-line photographs** *of these examples. Look for general similarities to yourself. Note that sub-types cause the differences in appearance between members of the same type.*

―――

## GOVERNMENT

> Secretary of State Warren Christopher
>   (Pres. Clinton cabinet)
> Supreme Court Justice Ruth Bader
>   Ginsburg

## ACTING

| | |
|---|---|
| Woody Allen | Stan Laurel |
| Pee Wee Herman | Bob Denver |
| Don Knotts | Lyle Lovett |
| Audrey Hepburn | Mia Farrow |
| Sandy Duncan | Shelly Duvall |
| Lily Tomlin | Calista Flockheart |

Janel Moloney ("The West Wing")

## SCIENCE

> Dr. Stephen Hawking, Cambridge physicist: a frail and famous scientist.

OTHER

Lesley Stahl ("60 Minutes")

*HISTORY (Rocine)*

Robert Louis Stevenson

*[I personally knew one of the above celebrities, and many in everyday life, which contributed to my understanding of the type.]*

Read the type, and if still confused see *Appendix* for the personal type identification request from my website: *DrStenbeck.net*

———

▶ *The type questionnaire pinpoints the major features of that type: if the celebrity examples are unhelpful, you may be an unusual variant (in which case ignore the celebrity issue and give yourself 7 points on Question 1).*

# *Atrophic Type Questionnaire*

*These questions describe the generic type, and not specifically you! If any question ever applied to you, then choose the True answer!*

---

*For Question 1 only:*

| | | |
|---|---|---|
| *A = True* | *B = Maybe* | *C = Untrue* |
| *15 points* | *7 points* | *1 point* |

1. Physically identify with celebrity example ____

---

*Others:*

| | | |
|---|---|---|
| *A = True* | *B = Maybe* | *C = Untrue* |
| *5 points* | *3 points* | *1 point* |

---

2. Usual height is close to:
   Males: 5'6—6'4   Females: 4'10—5'8   ____
3. Usual weight is close to:
   Males: 90—155   Females: 70—125   ____
4. Small muscles with little strength   ____
5. Exclusive, private, introverted   ____
6. Head may appear large compared
   to a slight body   ____
7. Hair is fine, thin, or oily; balding
   tendency   ____
8. Very difficult to gain weight   ____
9. Weak faith in God and religion   ____
10. High mental and creative abilities   ____
11. History of teeth weakness   ____
12. Prominent forehead   ____

13. Thin or frail body _____
14. Weak muscles _____
15. Receding lower jaw, small chin _____
16. Impatient _____
17. Weak bones, joints, and back _____
18. Great students, love to learn _____
19. Sunken face, long from large
forehead to chin, sloping jaw lines _____
20. Born to be a vegetarian or vegan _____
21. Wide mouth; thin upper lip, larger
lower lip; husky voice _____
22. Teeth large, white or gray, irregular _____
23. High intellect, intelligent, debaters _____
24. Abdomen, hollow, indented; almost
never have a pot-belly; narrow hips _____
25. Extremities thin, long, bony; may
have bow-legs _____
26. Have strong family ties _____
27. Aloof, awkward, or socially timid _____
28. Detail workers: science, authors,
accountancy, law, engineering, etc. _____
29. May be emotionally combative,
argumentative _____
30. Ears often odd-shaped, long, and thin _____
31. A thin, long, prominent nose with
pinched nostrils is usual _____
32. Introverted and passive _____
33. Skin moist or easily irritated; rosy
cheeks common (mostly females) _____
34. Markedly narrow, sunken, thin, chest;
some deformed rib structures; small
or no bust _____

35. Slow to anger (don't forgive easily if offended) _____
36. Tend to be withdrawn and moody _____
37. Easily charm the opposite sex _____
38. Have strong dislikes _____
39. Often skeptical _____
40. Pessimistic about the present _____
41. Optimistic about the future _____
42. Have strong will-power _____
43. May be arrogant and stubborn _____
44. Have little faith in others _____
45. Fine wrinkles, thin, fragile, skin _____
46. Often crave sex (or be addicted to it) _____
47. Disdainful or critical tendency _____
48. Sensitive to altitude and barometric changes _____
49. Have many health concerns _____
50. Dislike physical labor _____
51. Weak lungs; sinus, chronic infections, asthma common _____

▶ *The type questionnaire pinpoints the major features of that type: if the celebrity examples are unhelpful, you may be an unusual variant (in which case ignore the celebrity issue and give yourself 7 points on Question 1).*

_____

# Scoring
## For question #1:
A response: give 15 points = _____
B response: give 7 points = _____
C response: give 1 points = _____

## For questions #2—51:
A response: give 5 points = _____
B response: give 3 points = _____
C response: give 1 point = _____

*Total of the above points* = _____

## Interpretation
**136—245: PROBABLY Atrophic type**
*69—135: POSSIBLY Atrophic type*
*<69: NOT Atrophic type*

*Note –*

You already know something about this type from their public persona and appearance, whether from seeing them yourself or from the celebrity examples. Blend such insights with the type descriptions and the types of your family and friends to discern their presence in your midst!

Read the types, and if still confused you may choose to use the personal request for type identification from the Appendix or from my web site: *DrStenbeck.net*

———

# *The Atrophic Type*

*Rocine: "Atrophic, means un-nourished."*
*Food calcium and phosphorus, excessively*
*utilized in your metabolism, is invariably*
*deficient compared to other minerals. Your*
*overall mineral absorption is the poorest of all*
*types. You are a mental type, invariably*
*highly intelligent and intellectual.*

―――――

You are under-nourished because of genetic limitations in your metabolism making you sickly, bony, thin, and slight of build—you are the frailest of all people; a muscle sub-type may give you more strength. It is very difficult for you to gain weight. Your brain may be brilliant with a superior intellect, while in some it is latent.

▶ *I have known several members of your type who looked like holocaust survivors, an unhealthy way for you to be, yet, not unusual for some of you.*

Calcium absorption is very active and invariably excessive with spurts of bony growth in childhood causing you to be tall, frail, and ungainly. If such absorption falters you may be short and frail with an above-average intellect; if tall, you invariably have high intelligence and intellect. You often have a sunken chest or deformed rib-cage (also seen in the *marasmic*).

You may be beautiful or elegant like Audrey Hepburn and Calista Flockheart ("Ali McBeal") or intellectually handsome like Woody. The *atrophics* I have known are intellectual, reserved, diplomatic, and poised. You often have highly active phosphorus metabolism that enhances your intellect, intelligence, and potential for accomplishment as in Woody Allen and prior Secretary of State Warren Christopher (Clinton Administration).

You have pencil-thin bones and muscles: mostly, you cannot gain fat or be athletic. Your weak lungs cause inadequate oxygenation of lung tissues, asthma being a common sequeli.

▶ *For healing, you need to eat natural organic foods free from pesticides and chemicals, live in clean air, be vegetarian or vegan, and to eat dairy foods along with your type mineral foods.*

You have the most fragile health base of all types and need more preventive care than others. If anyone needs to live out of a health food store, it is you! Eating dairy foods benefits your health, so remember to eat them.

———

## Physical Similarity to Other Types

The *marasmic* type (Pres. George Bush, Sr., Vanessa Redgrave) is always tall, intelligent, thin or lean, and much stronger than the *atrophic*.

The *sillevitic* type (David Bowie, Carol Channing) is blonde or brunette, may look frail, and is more physically resilient compared to your type.

––––––

## Average Height and Weight

| | | |
|---|---|---|
| Males: | 5'6-6'4 | 90-155 pounds |
| Females: | 4'10-5'8 | 70-125 pounds |

––––––

# *Atrophic Type Description*

*The type description represents how you appear in everyday society. You may have a sub-type that alters parts of this description.*

The males may be over six feet (with some shorter like Woody Allen), whereas the females are usually of short to medium height.

*Head* —The head and forehead are large and may appear out of proportion to your slight body. The back-head is smaller.

*Hair* —The hair is thinning, brown or black, and often oily. In many males, the hair is thin and lifeless.

*Eyes* — You have blue, brown, or gray eyes.

*Ears* —Your ears are often odd-shaped, long, thin, and somewhat atypical looking (as in Calista and Audrey).

*Nose* — A thin, long, and prominent nose with pinched nostrils is usual.

*Face* — You typically show a long, narrow, and sunken face, from a large forehead to your long sloping jaws.

*Mouth, Lips and Voice* —Your wide mouth has thin lips, the lower lip is usually full and large. The voice is low-powered, quiet, weak, unique, and passive. You have a fine intellectual debating talent.

*Teeth* —Irregular calcium metabolism usually produces large, fragile, odd-shaped white teeth (requiring cosmetic dentistry).

*Skin* —Your skin is moist, fragile, sensitive, delicate, easily irritated, with fine wrinkles. A facial flush, or rosy cheeks, particularly in females, is indicative of lost body heat from trace mineral deficiencies or from a sluggish circulatory system; this poor health signal is corrected upon health recovery.

▶ *Many atrophic people have these facial features. I recall several men who were about 6'6 tall and several small frail females, all with small veins broken over their cheeks giving them the red flush. This flush may also come from allergies, which are common in this type.*

Note that the *sillevitic* may also undergo cheek flushing, but without the venous fragility, so study that type thoroughly. (Several carnivorous muscle types with parasympathetic nervous system dominance may also have a flushed complexion, but without the vascular fragility.)

*Neck* — The neck is usually long, gaunt, and lean.

*Muscles* — You cannot gain weight through weight-lifting, but may achieve a little strength.

*Chest* — You have a markedly narrow, sunken, and fragile chest, structural rib-cage abnormalities being common. There is little or no bust.

▶ *You have little muscle strength and are the weakest of all people. If able to do effective weight-lifting you are probably __not__ atrophic, more likely marasmic, neurogenic, medeic, or nervimotive.*

*Back and Shoulders* — Your back is long with square bony shoulders.

*Hips and Abdomen* —The abdomen is thin and indented, and your hips narrow. A protruding belly is impossible except in protein deficiency.

*Arms and Legs* —The extremities are thin, scrawny, long, and bony; you are often bow-legged or have knock-knees.

*Joints* — Your joints are weak and easily damaged.

————

## Atrophic Personality Traits

*If you are this type many, but not all, of the following characteristics are present—you may have overcome or moderated the negatives, but recognize that you once had several of them.*

# *Positive Qualities*

You may show any of the following traits:

- Very emotionally sensitive
- High intelligence and intellect
- Are optimistic about the future
- Charming with the opposite sex
- An assertive problem-solving mind
- High self-confidence and self-value
- Strong will power, optimistic about the future
- Are quiet, serene, brilliant, but held back by low vitality
- Have expertise in detailed mental work, law, medicine, literary, mathematics, science, accountancy, engineering, great scholars

# *Potential Challenges*

You tend to have low self-esteem and to be overly critical of others.

▶ *All people have some negative traits, but your brain tends to be aloof or combative, which may interfere with relationships and success. On the other hand, you are capable of being very charming to the opposite sex! One man I knew, seemed to have a harem around him all the time.*

You may have evolved from or not experienced these general faults, so do not dwell on them:

- Moody or depressed
- Lack faith or trust in God
- Often pessimistic about the present
- Tend to be gloomy, sad and withdrawn
- May have sexual addictions and cravings
- Aloof, demanding, combative, feisty tendency
- Are introverted, passive, unsociable, easily angered
- May seek revenge if slighted, combative, unforgiving
- Impatient, disdainful, stubborn tendency, prefer solitude
- Skeptical, timid, and awkward, strong dislikes, easily angered

▶ *If you relate to any of these challenges, doing something to overcome them serves your evolution.*

———

## Atrophic Stress Management

Your strong *mental* stress prevention gives you good defense against internalizing this stress into your stomach, adrenals, and immune system. *Emotional* stress prevention is not strong, and any of the above challenges may need help. *[If needing help managing these stresses, see my prior books.]*

———

# Love

You need a mate who is a thinker, mental, intellectual, passionate, creative, vegetarian, and highly sexual. You are attracted to intelligent types.

———

# Talents and Vocations

You have high intelligence and intellect, and are great students. You love to study and often accomplish high academic honors in the sciences and professions. Some of you may be uneducated and found in any work requiring good mental-power. The type information cannot predict what or who you will become, but you are capable of bringing creative excellence to whatever you do in life.

**Abilities** - *Scientific, law, philosophy, literary*

Your talents are mental and intellectual. Your powerful brain is brilliant, skilled, creative, and painstaking. You are interested in education and science. Some *atrophics* become great writers and authors, like Robert Louis

Stephenson. I have known you as doctors, writers, scientists, professors, many more in the arts and sciences, and still others with unrealized potential.

▶ *Rocine: "Atrophics have more phosphorus than the calciferic, hence are more active mentally."*

[*Calciferics* themselves are mental giants!]

**Inabilities** - *Physical labor, executive or managerial*

You disdain physical labor, and are too physically and emotionally sensitive to be an effective manager.

———

## Atrophic Health Problems

You are environmentally sensitive, and this sensitivity superimposed on your weak genetics or poor immunity causes life-long health problems. Eating correct food combinations and organic foods is critical for your health along with removing environmental toxins from your body (see later diet section).

▶ *Rocine: "To stay healthy you should become a relentless advocate of natural foods and healing methods—medicine and drugs kill you. Holistic doctors and natural medicines are your savior."*

When sick, you may experience any of these health problems:

*Allergies* — It is important to identify and avoid your common allergies to air and water impurities, household chemicals, environmental toxins, electrical circuits, GMO and other foods, and so on.

*Lungs* — A weak brain medulla predisposes you to asthma. Your weakest organ, the lungs are often associated with ribcage abnormalities.

*Chronic Infections* — Lung, sinus, and intestinal infections are common.

*Bones and Joints* — You have weak and vulnerable joints, bones, ligaments, and tendons, and you may be arthritic.

*Digestive System* — This system is inefficient and liable to constipation, diarrhea, indigestion, and dysfunction.

*Nervous System* —You deal with stress well, but headaches are common.

*Skin* —Sores, irritations, discharges, skin imperfections, and healing problems are common.

▶ *Some of you are so sick and environmentally sensitive that you can hardly live a normal life or live in the average home because of: paint, carpets, chemicals, climate, barometric pressures, temperature changes, and electrical wiring—you need to leave the city and live close to mother nature.*

————

## *Atrophic Acid/Alkaline Factor*

*[See Chapter 3 for details on this subject, along with the common symptoms found with people of different nervous system dominance.]*

For your health and healing, the genetics of your nervous system require attention to the acidity or alkalinity of your daily food intake. You are born with an **acid constitution** requiring a predominantly *alkaline-ash* food intake (for acid/alkaline balance). Ash refers to the mineral ash left in your body after metabolizing foods. The *atrophic* autonomic nervous system genetics are *sympathetic* dominant. Construct this approximate ratio of food selections (for your daily food intake).

> *80% Fruits, salads, vegetables*
> *20% Proteins, carbohydrates*

---

## The Atrophic Spiritual Factor

*Skip this paragraph if uninterested in a philosophical perspective on your body type!*

▶ *Rocine: "The soul chooses the body type."*

If as souls, we choose the brain and body type to spend a lifetime in, it could be to learn certain spiritual lessons related to perfecting ourselves, and our humanity (in God's eyes). What lessons does the type bring to you? Only you can really decide what they are. You know your weaknesses and faults. You know things about yourself that Victor Rocine could never get from his research subjects when he first wrote about types. So search your mind for the answers. Each type has discrete life lessons, spiritual goals, etc., and some of yours probably are:

*Faith* — This is perhaps your most important challenge: you often feel separated from God (and have little faith) and need to work on this aspect.

*Health* — Being this type and living in a weak and sickly physical body along with a very intelligent and creative brain, serves your evolution in some particular way.

*Accomplishment* — Work on developing your magnificent left-brain, and possibly manifesting excellence or greatness in your field of activity.

*People* — Being more giving of yourself to loved ones, is a challenge because you become lost in your thoughts. Work on it. You are powerful mentally, but it is important to become more emotionally vulnerable.

*Arrogance* — You may need humility lessons to accept you are no better than other people in God's eyes! Become humble; control your ego imbalance, arrogance, and combativeness. Therapy helps.

*Impatience* — Overcoming this trait requires you develop patience with those of inferior intellect!

*Judgmental, Critical* — Negative judgment of others is a fault.

*Sexual Addiction* — Use willpower to moderate this problem, males particularly; heal any childhood negative sexual programming.

▶ *You are unconcerned as to whether people like you or not. You may see the above personality traits as strengths! Have more harmonious interaction with others and perhaps achieve greater spiritual evolution! If you relate to any of the above challenges, overcoming them serves your evolution.*

———

## An Atrophic Story...

At age 16, Jeanette's parents had despaired about her diet, health, and behaviors. Jeanette had chronic ill-health of body and mind. Her body was frail, weak, under-nurtured, and malfunctioning in many organ systems. The net result was hypoglycemia, with no energy, little hormone production, and a lack of joy and motivation.

Dietary evaluation showed calcium deficiencies requiring: kelp, cheddar cheese, turnip greens, almonds, and Brewer's yeast. She also showed deficits in phosphorus foods: brewer's yeast, whole wheat, and seeds (pumpkin, sunflower, squash, and sesame).

Her energy and health quickly improved after following the type diet.

———

# *Atrophic Type Mineral Food Needs*

*Apply this mineral data to the diet following the Thin type descriptions.*

## Excessive Foods:
- *Chlorine (salted, junk)*
- *Nitrogen (animal)*

## Deficient Foods:
- *Phosphorus*
- *Calcium*
- *Potassium*
- *Sodium (unsalted, non-junk)*
- *Trace Minerals*
- *Carbon (carbohydrates)*
- *Nitrogen (vegetable)*

*These deficient minerals are common deficiencies in your type, and predispose you to ill-health. If ill, be sure to use these lists with your daily food intake. If not ill, eat from the food lists 3-4 days weekly for health maintenance.*

*All food lists are in descending order of concentration and value to you; choose servings of foods in the upper half of each list first! One serving is ½ cup.*

# *Excessive Foods -*

*Chlorine* is easily absorbed and usually excessive in your type, contributing to a gaunt lean body and to a negative emotional state. Avoid processed foods and common salt!

*Nitrogen (animal source)* is excessive, a major cause of acidity, and illnesses from red meat intake (minimize other meats, poultry, fish, and eggs).

▶ *If ill or diseased nitrogen imbalance (protein) is often a significant healing factor. If ill, eating lamb 1-2 times weekly is healthy for you in restoring protein balance; the lamb is then discontinued.*

―――――

# *Deficient Foods -*

*If ill or diseased, eating these mineral foods is important for your healing.*

*Phosphorus* is often deficient in your tissues because of brain exhaustion and intense nervous system activity; you are always thinking, planning, and worrying about everything in your life—especially your health. If ill or diseased, a phosphorus deficiency is probably an important factor. (Eating phosphorus foods and taking

*Phosfood* tablets made by Standard Process Laboratories is valuable in this instance.)

*Calcium* absorption is poor and a common deficiency; you need daily calcium supplements and liberal dairy foods (on which you thrive). You may need to take a 'lactase' supplement with dairy foods.

*Potassium* is a common deficiency in your type. It is a dominant element in your tissues and is vital to the health of your muscles, heart, brain, and to all cells. If ill or diseased, potassium supplements are often a significant healing factor.

*Sodium* in food form (unsalted) is deficient in your type. Such sodium foods, needed for all body types, help eliminate calcium deposition in joints, arteries, and soft tissues. If ill or diseased, an important healing factor is to stop eating fast foods, lose the salt shaker, and to eat *unsalted* sodium foods instead.

*Trace minerals* become deficient in your type due to emotional stress or poor digestion and absorption. All types need trace minerals, especially you! Liquid sources are best.

*Carbon* is deficient in your tissues and needed for building more flesh. For health, increase your intake of complex carbohydrate (starches, whole grain cereals, breads) and minimize intake of simple sugars (candy, cakes, sweets, white sugar products). You may need to build more fat on your body to help your healing.

*Nitrogen* (vegetable sources) is often deficient. Emphasize in your diet vegetarian proteins like legumes (peas, beans), soy, seeds, nuts, and pasta, and if ill take a protein drink.

*[See the Appendix for descriptions of mineral functions in the body.]*

▶ *Approximate your food ratios. On any particular day, it does not matter if one meal is mostly alkaline and another mostly acid—just try to balance it out for the day! If you make a mistake, try again tomorrow. It is a subjective call that you make. What you do over time makes the difference to your health.*

---

---

## *Minimize* *Excessive Foods*

**Chlorine** *(salted, junk food):*
 *0-1 servings/week*

*Salt, all fast foods, packaged foods, canned and frozen foods, soy sauce, all preserved meats (cured, smoked, canned and luncheon meats), sauces (barbecue, catsup, etc.), dill pickles, sauerkraut, bouillon cubes, peanut butter, potato chips, etc., salted nuts, crackers, canned or packaged soups, processed cheeses, commercial salad dressings, meat tenderizers.*

*Note - If underweight, also minimize these chlorine foods: 0-2 times/week*

*Fish, alfalfa, goat brown cheese, egg white, butter, rye, spinach, ripe olives.*

**Nitrogen**: *0-1 times /month*

*Meats, poultry*

---

▶ *You are the only type genetically destined to be vegan or vegetarian: another type may choose to become so, but for you it is a necessity.*

## *Eat*
## *Deficient Foods*

### *Phosphorus, Potassium, Sodium:*
*1-2 servings/day*

*Kelp, milk, goat milk, seeds (pumpkin, squash, sesame, sunflower), rice bran, cheese (except Brie, Roquefort, Swiss), brewer's yeast, whole wheat, Brazil nuts, soybeans, dulse, blackstrap molasses, raisins, parsley, almonds.*

### *Calcium:* *1-2 servings/day*

*Kelp, cheese (cottage, cheddar), turnip greens, carob flour, collard leaves, almonds, brewer's yeast, parsley, dandelion greens, Brazil nuts, watercress, dried figs, yogurt, beet greens, whole wheat, milk, seeds (and green vegetable juices).*

### *Trace Minerals:* *1-2 servings/day*

*Ginger, rice, oats, pecans, pineapples, kelp, brewer's yeast, rye, dry split peas, blackstrap molasses, seeds (pumpkin, squash, sun flower), Brazil nuts, peanuts, rice, oat straw and alfalfa teas.*

## *Eat…*

**Carbon** *(complex carbohydates): As desired*
*Starches, grains, breads, sweet fruit*

**Nitrogen** *(vegetable):*
*Soy, peas, seeds, nuts, pasta, and spirulina:*
*2-3 servings/day*
*Organic eggs, fresh fish:  0-2 times/week*
*Be sure to avoid eating any allergic foods.*

**Vegetable Protein Drink:** *(once daily)*
*Take a high protein, high calorie, powdered*
*vegetable protein supplement: about 20-30 gm.,*
*in juice or milk, once daily, on an empty*
*stomach; drink it slowly over thirty or more*
*minutes for better digestion.*

Note - *The food recommendations are for the*
*generic type. Additionally, you may need from a*
*holistic healer or nutritionist something more*
*specific for your individuality. Eat any healthy foods*
*you desire, but be sure to include the type foods in*
*your daily choices.*

# *Atrophic Nutritional Supplements*

- **Multi-Vitamin-Minerals** —
  *2 capsules daily*

- **Potassium** —*99 mg/day* ``

- **Lecithin** — *About 1,300 mg/three
  times weekly*

- **Evening Primrose or Flaxseed
  Oil** —*1 soft-gel/day*

- **Calcium/Magnesium** —
  *About 600 mg. calcium (combined with
  magnesium), twice daily, combined with
  betaine hydrochloride and vitamin D*

- **Herbs** —
  *Brain detox – Vervain or Valerian Root
  Organ detox – Milk Thistle or Strawberry
  Leaf (one capsule, twice daily with food for
  one month; then one, three times weekly).*

- **Other** —
  *Chlorophyll, blue-green algae, green
  magma, alfalfa (Take as directed.)*

# *Important Atrophic Health Concerns*

Be sure to take the above supplements if you have ill-health. If in good health (unlikely) take them at least 3-4 times weekly.

Genetically you are a *partial or complete* vegetarian. Generally, the more meat you eat the sicker you become. If ill, eating lamb 2-3 times weekly accelerates healing, any meat craving is a protein deficiency that disappears with protein balance. (See the Thin type Food Guide.)

---

## *ATROPHIC FOOD GUIDE*

### *Aim for -*
80% Fruits, salads, vegetables
20% Proteins, carbohydrates
*and*
90% Raw food diet
### **You thrive on dairy foods**
*(use raw milk products if possible)*
*Take the recommended supplements.*

---

▶ *Rocine: "You thrive on dairy foods and they are important for your health, especially raw pasteurized goat milk."*

———

## Atrophic Fat Loss

Invariably, for your health and healing, you need to gain fat by increasing your daily calorie intake with healthy fatty foods, and a high-calorie protein drink.

———

# *Thin Types*
# *General Food Guide*

*(Vegetarian or Semi-Vegetarian)*

# *Important Note*

———

The Food Guide addresses the <u>Acid-Alkaline</u> aspect of your food intake, along with the <u>Type Mineral</u> factor presented throughout this book. It does <u>not</u> necessarily address calories or other dietary factors that may be pertinent to your personal health needs whether medical or appropriate for some other dietary need. So use your common sense and just include the factors described here with whatever healthy dietary choices you usually make.

For other nutrient information, consult with nutritional books or with holistic nutritional doctors. I particularly recommend the advice of Andrew Weil, M.D.

———

# *General Food Guide*

*This chapter presents a general Food Guide, upon which you superimpose the nutritional information from your type chapter.*

———

## *Meat/Flesh Intake*

Most muscle types should limit red meat to once or less weekly, while eggs, lamb, fish, or poultry are excellent in moderation. If ill or diseased, be sure to eat daily, one or two servings from each *deficient minerals* list. If not ill, eat them at least three times weekly for health maintenance. If this diet is similar to your present diet, but healing is sluggish, then:

- Decrease your carbohydrate and protein intake by about one-third
- Increase your fruit, salad, and vegetable intake by about one-third
- Consult with a holistic doctor, preferably one versed in nutritional and emotional evaluation

———

## Over-Acid or Over-Alkaline?

Just as a log of wood burned in your fireplace leaves a mineral-ash, food ash refers to the minerals remaining after metabolizing foods in your tissues:

- Fruits, vegetables **alkalinize** tissues
- Proteins, carbohydrates **acidify** tissues

## Usually You Are Over-Acid Due To:

- Excessive intake of dairy foods
- Excessive intake of proteins and carbohydrates
- Deficient intake of fruits, salads and vegetables
- Accumulated metabolic waste-acids (from years of eating excessive acid-ash foods, meats and carbohydrates, and from lack of exercise)
- You need to estimate the ratio of foods eaten. Generally, eat the following *approximate* ratios for your health:

> **80% Alkaline-ash** foods *(fruits, salads, vegetables)*
> **20% Acid-ash** foods *(complex carbohydrates like starches, grains, cereals, breads, flour products; and proteins)*

Approximate your food ratios. On any particular day, it does not matter if one meal is mostly alkaline, and another mostly acid—just try to balance it out for the day! If you get it wrong, try again tomorrow. It is a subjective call that you make, and it is what you do over weeks, months, or years that make the difference—not on any one or two days.

————

## *Important*

- Minimize white sugar and alcohol intake.
- If desired, interchange lunches for dinners.
- Never eat foods you are allergic to, no matter what I recommend; if allergic, or suspect a food allergy, eliminate it and substitute from your type mineral lists.
- Eat the right foods 80-90% of the time and the Food Guide will work for you; unlike some types you do not have to live out of a health food store (although such foods are healthier for you).

► *Observe the excessive minerals in your type chapter, and be sure to eat one or two servings from the deficient list daily (or, several times weekly).*

Finally, in addition to your body type needs, other holistic healing matters also need your attention. I strongly suggest that you refer to my web site and earlier books for that information: *DrStenbeck.net*

———

## *Important*

- Minimize white sugar and alcohol intake.

- If desired, interchange lunches for dinners.

- Never eat foods you are allergic to no matter what is recommended; if allergic or suspect a food allergy, eliminate it and substitute from your type mineral lists.

- Eat the right foods 80-90% of the time and the *Food Guide* will work for you.

- You may have allergies to wheat, corn, other grains, sugar, alcohol, and milk (examine your body reactions to these foods for fatigue, sinusitis, joint pain, skin rash, and gastro-intestinal reactions). Note that the *atrophic* type *requires* dairy foods for health and healing.

- Living out of a health food store is unnecessary (although such foods are healthier for you). If you want dietary

perfection in your healing efforts, eat
organic foods (from a health food store).

In addition to your body type needs other
holistic healing matters also need your
attention. I suggest that you refer to my web
site and earlier books for that information:
*DrStenbeck.net*

———

# *Thin Types*
# *General Food Guide*

*[Superimpose the nutritional information from your Type Chapter into this Food Guide.]*

## *Breakfast*

---

FRUIT *salad, fresh (with citrus fruit) and* <u>*protein*</u>*: yogurt, kefir, milk, cheeses, or raw seeds or nuts — 3+ times/week; or*

CEREALS *(whole grain), fruit, seeds, and nuts as desired — 2+ times/week; or*

EGGS *(1-2) with lettuce, tomato, veges, non-wheat toast — 0-3 times/week; or*

OTHER *choices — 0-1 times/week*

### <u>*Daily Liquids*</u>

*Coffee, teas — 0-1 cups*
*Pure water, citrus, fruit, or vegetable juices, soups, other — as desired*
*Wheat is a common allergy: avoid white breads; eat sour dough, millet, or oat breads instead.*
*Note: For in-between snacks, have fruit or vegetables, with seeds or nuts.*

---

# *Lunch*

*SALADS*, mixed green, with <u>*protein*</u> *(cheese, soy, seeds, egg, etc.) Dressing: virgin olive oil and vinegar, low-fat dressings — 3-5 times weekly; and/or*

*VEGETABLES with salad (and a <u>protein</u>: yogurt, cottage cheese...) — 1-3 times/week; or*

*FRUIT salad (like breakfast)*
*— 1-2 times/week; or*

*SANDWICH, whole grains, cheese and /or other non-flesh <u>protein</u>; small salad*
*— 0-2 times/week; or*

*OTHER choices*
*— 0-1 times/week*

*\* Other oils less ideal; soybean oil is a common allergen; minimize commercial dressings.*

# *Dinner*

*VEGETARIAN meals: include legumes, tofu, cheese, cottage cheese, seeds, nuts, egg, etc. (and/or salad) — 2+ times/week; or*

*POULTRY/FISH (3-6 oz.), salad and/or vegetables — 0-2 times/week; or*

*WHOLE GRAIN PASTA, cooked (barley, rice, millet, etc.), and salad/or vegetables — 0-2 times/week; or*

*OTHER choices — 1-2 times weekly*

*DESSERTS: Fruits, fresh or low-sugar desserts — as desired*

*Note: Be sure to include one or more selections from your type food lists in your daily food intake.*

*Note.* If *vegetarian* substitute flesh proteins with seeds, nuts, legumes, and other vegetables. You are vulnerable to being protein deficient so be careful to eat sufficient proteins and/or include a daily protein drink!

# *Food Guide Notes*

*Steamed Vegetables* — Minerals are lost in the boiling of vegetables, so steaming or wok cooking is best.

*Food Combinations* — Eating proteins at the same meal with starches often results in indigestion, gas or constipation (as does eating fruit and starch together). For those of you with weak digestive systems, watch how this or other inharmonious combinations may be affecting you.

*Periodic Detox Dieting* — If you over-indulge in acid-ash foods, you need occasional elimination diets for tissue waste-acid removal, supervised by a nutritional doctor.

*Minimize* —
- Plums, cranberries, and their juices
- Commercial, sugared, and fatty salad dressings
- Red meats, processed meats, wines, alcohol, and milk
- Coffee, white sugar, fructose, and chemical sugar substitutes
- Exposure to drugs, environmental chemicals, pesticides
- Avoid eating allergic foods

*Healthy Weight* — You have a good ability to lose and control weight by following the Food Guide instructions. If you gain weight, the most common reason is liver or kidney irritation due to food allergies or negative emotions—the key is to eat non-allergic foods. The *atrophic and marasmic* types usually need to gain weight. (Obviously, if you have a medical condition that contradicts this advice, do not change your diet!)

———

## In Conclusion

It may be difficult to discern your type from the *marasmic and sillevitic* types. Study them well and you will see the differences.

———

# *Appendix*

## *Brief Extracts from*
## *The 22 Unique Body Types*

*A. Types / Minerals*      *48*

*B. Researchers*      *52*

*C. Genetics, Types, and Diet*      *54*

*D. Help identifying your body type,*
*     with Dr. Stenbeck*      *57*

*E. On-line Health Consultation*
*     with Dr. Stenbeck*      *60*

*F. Notes*      *61*

*Appendix A*

# *Types*
## *(Brief extract)*

Type comes from 'typus' meaning an image or impression, the study of types being called typology.

▶ *Rocine: "A combination of mental and structural features is consistently found in people of the same type."*

Rocine wrote that all types are a mixture of positive and negative qualities. He based his work on the biochemical individuality of our *mineral* absorption and utilization. Of course, all minerals are absorbed, but he postulated that different types of people *selectively* absorb certain minerals, to a greater or lesser extent, requiring specific mineral foods for their enhanced health and healing.

▶ *The type information cannot predict what or who you will become, or how successful or not, but your type is capable of bringing a creative excellence to whatever you do in life. If your type has negative qualities that you disagree with, remember that they are only tendencies and may or may not manifest in you.*

This book enlarges on Rocine's premise (early 1900's), integrated with the later research of Herbert Sheldon, M.D., Ph.D., at Harvard University (1930's), along with my fifty years of observations and experience with this subject.

Comparing your shared physical (and sometimes psychological) descriptions with the Celebrity Lists further assists the identification of your type. It is not that you will look exactly like, or be a twin to, any particular celebrity. Look closely at a celebrity's features: face, profile, height, weight, head, etc. If you know something about their talents, beliefs, success and failure spheres, health and weight challenges, attitudes and behaviors, etc., then you get clues as to what your type may be.

———

## Understanding Types and Sub-Types

Each of us has a clearly discernible dominant type. Visualize the celebrity examples from movies, politics, sports, the arts and public life, and try to identify with their physical features. Look for similar features, remembering that you will not recognize all attributes in yourself. You are not looking for your twin!

The sub-type issue is the main reason people of the same major type can look so different. Remember that a type description does not characterize you exactly, but depicts your individual variant of a type.

▶ *The type questionnaire pinpoints the major features of that type: if the celebrity examples are unhelpful, you may be an unusual variant (in which case ignore the celebrity issue and give yourself 7 points on Question 1).*

---

## *Minerals*

Minerals are essential life nutrients that accelerate enzyme and chemical reactions and provide a basis for your body typing. Although found in all tissues, different minerals tend to be concentrated in certain organs, their presence or absence contributing to the healing of such tissues; e.g., zinc accelerates prostate healing; calcium and manganese promote bone, joint and connective tissue healing.

Specific foods nurture each type, some people needing meats for their health others needing a vegetarian diet. A high potassium diet nurtures one person, while another needs high sulfur, calcium, zinc, or another mineral.

## Mineral Digestion and Absorption

Compared to vitamins, minerals are *difficult* to digest, absorb, and utilize. In people with strong digestive systems, this aspect may not be important. The following factors should be in place for optimal mineral metabolism:

1. Stomach Hydrochloric Acid Production
2. Parathyroid Hormone Balance
3. Organ Toxic Metal and Chemical Removal
   *[See details in <u>The 22 Unique Body Types</u>.]*

———

## Total Body Healing

Note that from a holistic healing perspective, in addition to minerals and type information, the following healing factors are necessary:

> *Nutrient Balance*
> *Mental Balance*
> *Emotional Balance*
> *Spiritual Balance*
> *Detoxifying Integrity*

The above factors are all important to your total healing especially if you are interested in self-healing (see my earlier books).

———

*Appendix B*

# *Researchers*
## *(Brief extract)*

The predominant workers in this area of human individuality from around 1880's to the 1960's are Herbert Sheldon, M.D., Ph.D., Roger Williams, Ph.D., and Victor Rocine, D.Sc.

Much information on Sheldon's research exists on-line and in medical psychology libraries; for interested readers there are other lines of research published in the last century. This present book is primarily about Rocine's body types.

## *Herbert Sheldon M.D., Ph.D.*

In contrast to Rocine, Sheldon at Harvard University in the 1930's was trained in the scientific method and did painstaking research and publishing on human individuality. In comparing his findings with Rocine's work, a direct putative correlation is visible.

## *Roger J. Williams, Ph.D.*

Another significant researcher in human individuality is the renowned scientist and biochemist, Roger J. Williams. He demon-strated that different people have varying levels of nutrients, enzymes, and other metabolic chemicals in their bloodstreams.

▶ *Williams's research firmly expands on the premise of individual nutritional needs in human beings. If interested in his research, I highly recommend his book <u>Biochemial Individuality</u>.*

## *Victor Rocine, D.Sc.*

Note that when a negative feature is indicated, say neurotic tendencies, all members of the type are <u>not</u> that way; it is a type tendency reported by Rocine.

Rocine studied type-related diseases finding links between mineral and dietary factors with individual types and their diseases. In each body type, one or more dominant minerals are preferentially absorbed and utilized over other minerals.

He recognized discrete body types from their physical appearance finding genetically based mineral dominance to be the determining feature. He also correlated their physical features with psychological characteristics.

―――

*Appendix C*

# Genetics, Types, and Diet
### *(Brief extract)*

This section deals with how nervous system genetics helps determine your eating choices for health: you are either born to be a predominant meat eater, a partial or complete vegetarian, or something between the two. The genetic factor determining this dietary aspect is the *sympathetic and parasympathetic* components of your central nervous system. This represents a basic factor in eating for health.

This chapter helps you understand your dietary inheritance, although instinctively, you may already have arrived there!

- If born **sympathetic** dominant you are *genetically acid*, desiring a predominantly *vegetarian* diet for your health (about 70% fruit, salad, vegetables to 30% proteins and carbohydrates).

- If born **parasympathetic** dominant you are *genetically alkaline*, desiring a predominantly *carnivorous* diet for your health (about 70% proteins, carbohydrates to 30% fruits, salads, vegetables). Few of you ever choose to become vegetarian because of the difficulty in satisfying your protein needs without meats.

- If born ***intermediate*** dominant you may eat food groups with little concern for the acid/alkaline factor. However, after age 40, you need a semi-vegetarian diet for healthy eating.

———

## *Chart of Relative Nervous System Dominance*

In the following Chart, if you relate to many of the symptoms on one side you probably have that nervous system dominance; relating to both sides indicates *Intermediate* dominance.

### *If Vegetarian (Over-acid)* --
*Eat 70% fruits, salads, vegetables*
*And 30% proteins, carbohydrates*

### *If Carnivore  (Over-alkaline)* --
*Eat 70% proteins, carbohydrates*
*And 30% fruits, salads, vegetables*

### *If Intermediate* --
*Eat 50:50 of acid and alkaline-ash foods*

Make an *approximate* estimate of your daily acid and alkaline food intake (such ratios varying from type to type).

———

# Symptoms of Relative
# Genetic Dominance

| *Vegetarians*<br>*(Over-acid)* | *Carnivores*<br>*(Over-alkaline)* |
|---|---|
| *Sympathetic*<br>*Dominance* | *Parasympathetic*<br>*Dominance* |
| *little or no flesh desire* | *desire flesh* |
| *easily constipated* | *rarely constipated* |
| *slow digestion* | *fast digestion* |
| *easily dehydrated* | *not dehydrated* |
| *strong thirst* | *low thirst* |
| *pale face* | *flushed face* |
| *high pulse after food* | *slow pulse after food* |
| *easy gag reflex* | *slow gag reflex* |
| *cool dry skin* | *moist warm skin* |
| *nervous stomach* | *calm stomach* |
| *little eyelid blinking* | *much blinking* |
| *nervous tendency* | *mostly calm* |
| *slower healing* | *faster healing* |
| *low oxygen-uptake* | *good oxygen-uptake* |
| *easily breathless* | *seldom breathless* |
| *insomnia common* | *sleep easier* |
| *few muscle cramps* | *some night cramps* |
| *calcium deposits rare* | *get calcium deposits* |

## *Appendix D*

## **Help Identifying your Body Type with Dr. Stenbeck**

If you desire help in identifying your body type, follow these instructions, and answer the questionnaire. For further information and fees, send me an email from page one of the website:

### *DrStenbeck.net*

First name: _____

Country of birth: _____

*Upload photos and send to the above website:*

- Head and shoulders: front and side views

- Full body: front and side views

- Also 1-2 teenage views

- If possible, casual photos of mother, father, siblings

MY TYPE CLASS MAY BE: _____

(Thin, Muscle, or Fat)

AGE          -          _____

HEIGHT     -          _____ feet/inches

MY WEIGHT -          _____ pounds

Heaviest at age:          _____

- Lightest as adult: _____

- Estimate age 15: _____

VISION - Excellent  Average        Poor:

HAIR -   Natural color: _____

   - Thin/thick? _____

   - balding? _____

SKIN  - Quality: _____

   - History of acne, boils, other:

_____

_____

TEETH     - Strong          Weak      Dentures

          - Cavity history: Many      Moderate   Few

MUSCLES  - Strong        Average    Weak

      Sports played _____

JOINTS    - Strong        Average    Weak

HEALTH - Childhood diseases?

_____

_____

- Adult diseases?

_____

## AVERAGE DIET

- Beef _____ (times/week)

 - Poultry _____ (times/week)

 - Fish _____ (times/week)

 - Eggs _____ (times/week)

 - Water _____ (glasses/day):

 - Vegetarian? Vegan? _____

 - Other? _____

 - Did your childhood diet differ? _____

*The above will help me know who you are! I will send you a follow-up questionnaire for further help in identifying your body type.*

*Appendix E*

## **On-line Health Consultation with Dr. Stenbeck**

For further information, or to comment on this book, or to receive a response on any health issue from a holistic viewpoint, send an email inquiry from page one of my website:

### *DrStenbeck.net*

Following that, I will suggest further healing needs, which we may pursue with an on-line consult.

———

*Appendix F*

## *Notes*

See my book <u>*The 22 Unique Body Types,*</u> available at the usual online source, for further information and details on all of the 22 Types. The Appendix in that book has more information about:

*Mineral Functions and Food Sources*

*Further Reading*

———

www.ingramcontent.com/pod-product-compliance
Lightning Source LLC
Chambersburg PA
CBHW071229280526
45787CB00002B/852